THE FLAVORFUL HYPERTENSION DIET COOKBOOK

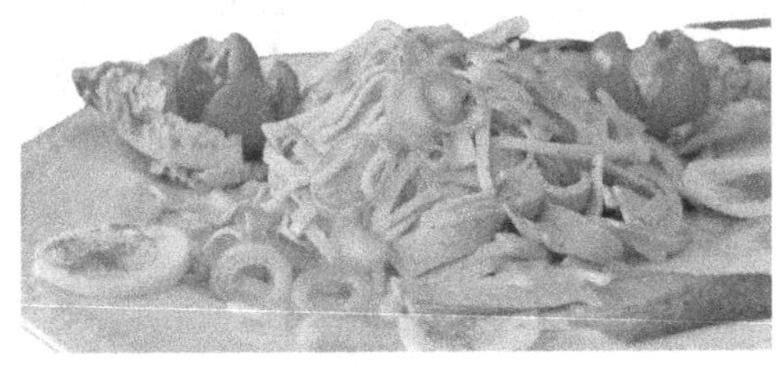

Savor The Symphony Of Health With Delicious Recipes For Managing High Blood Pressure

OLIVIA TRIMWELL

Copyright © 2023 by OLIVIA TRIMWELL

All rights reserved.

TABLE OF CONTENT

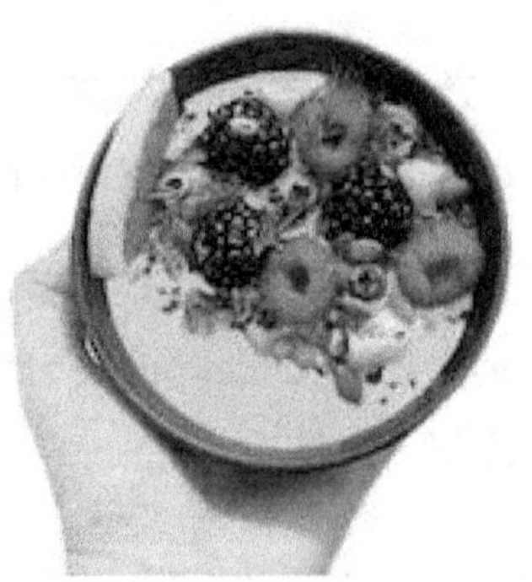

Introduction

In the hustle of present day lifestyles, Kate determined herself grappling with hypertension, a silent threat that crept into her day by day life. Doctors prescribed medicines, however the side consequences had been daunting, and the possibility of an entire life dependency left her disheartened. Desperate for an opportunity, Kate stumbled upon The Flavorful Hypertension Diet Cookbook, a beacon promising a route to fitness via scrumptious, heart-pleasant meals.

As she delved into the pages, Kate located a culinary adventure that now not handiest tantalized her taste buds but additionally provided a lifeline. The cookbook's recipes had been a symphony of vibrant flavors and healthful elements, meticulously curated to fight hypertension. Each dish appeared extra like a gastronomic journey than a scientific prescription.

Embracing the cookbook's teachings, Kate overhauled her weight loss plan, bidding farewell to processed ingredients weighted down with hidden sodium. Fresh herbs, colorful greens, and heart-healthful grains took center level in her kitchen. The transformative effect turned into gradual however profound. Kate's blood strain began to stabilize, and the incessant throbbing in her temples diminished into a distant memory.

The cookbook have become her depended on accomplice, guiding her through the art of conscious consuming. Kate's adventure from high blood pressure's clutches became not just about numbers on a scientific chart; it changed into a holistic transformation. She radiated newfound energy, her smile reflecting the colourful, nutrient-rich meals she now savored.

The Flavorful Hypertension Diet Cookbook had now not handiest rescued Kate from the grip of hypertension but had empowered her to savor existence with zest, proving that on occasion, the most potent medicine lies not in a tablet but at the plate earlier than you.

"The Flavorful Hypertension Diet Cookbook" is a complete manual designed to cope with the important difficulty of coping with high blood stress through a carefully curated and flavorful dietary technique. This cookbook goes past the traditional perception of restrictive diets, aiming to redefine the manner people perceive and interact with their nutritional choices. As high blood strain, or high blood pressure, remains a established fitness difficulty globally, expertise and enforcing an powerful nutritional method becomes paramount. This cookbook seeks to empower individuals with a numerous variety of delicious recipes that no longer handiest cater to their taste buds however additionally make a contribution to a more healthy way of life.

The importance of dealing with high blood strain thru a balanced food regimen can not be overstated. Hypertension is a leading danger element for numerous cardiovascular sicknesses, stroke, and different fitness complications. The incidence of this circumstance underscores the urgency of adopting proactive measures to manipulate and save you its unfavorable consequences. A balanced food plan plays a pivotal role on this enterprise, presenting a natural and sustainable method to retaining most fulfilling blood strain ranges.

The nutritional selections we make at once have an effect on our standard fitness, and inside the case of high blood pressure, they are able to both exacerbate or alleviate the circumstance. A weight loss plan rich in sodium, processed foods, and saturated fats can contribute to elevated blood pressure levels, while a eating regimen emphasizing whole ingredients, lean proteins, and nutrient-dense ingredients has been proven to have a effective impact. The incorporation of fruits, vegetables, whole grains, and lean proteins facilitates modify blood strain, lessen irritation, and guide universal cardiovascular fitness.

"The Flavorful Hypertension Diet Cookbook" recognizes the demanding situations individuals face while trying to adopt a heart-wholesome weight loss program and pursuits to bridge the space between nutritious and delicious. By imparting a numerous array of recipes that prioritize taste with out compromising on health advantages, the cookbook seeks to make the adventure toward dealing with high blood pressure an enjoyable and sustainable one.

The cookbook does not suggest for a one-length-fits-all approach; instead, it encourages a customized and bendy dietary plan that incorporates man or woman preferences and dietary regulations. This flexibility is essential in fostering lengthy-time period adherence to a heart-wholesome life-style, as rigid diets often cause frustration and abandonment.

In end, "The Flavorful Hypertension Diet Cookbook" introduces a refreshing angle on handling excessive blood strain via the lens of fun and nourishing meals. By highlighting the importance of a balanced food plan in high blood pressure management, the cookbook empowers readers to take control of their fitness even as savoring the wealthy and diverse flavors that a heart-healthful way of life can offer.

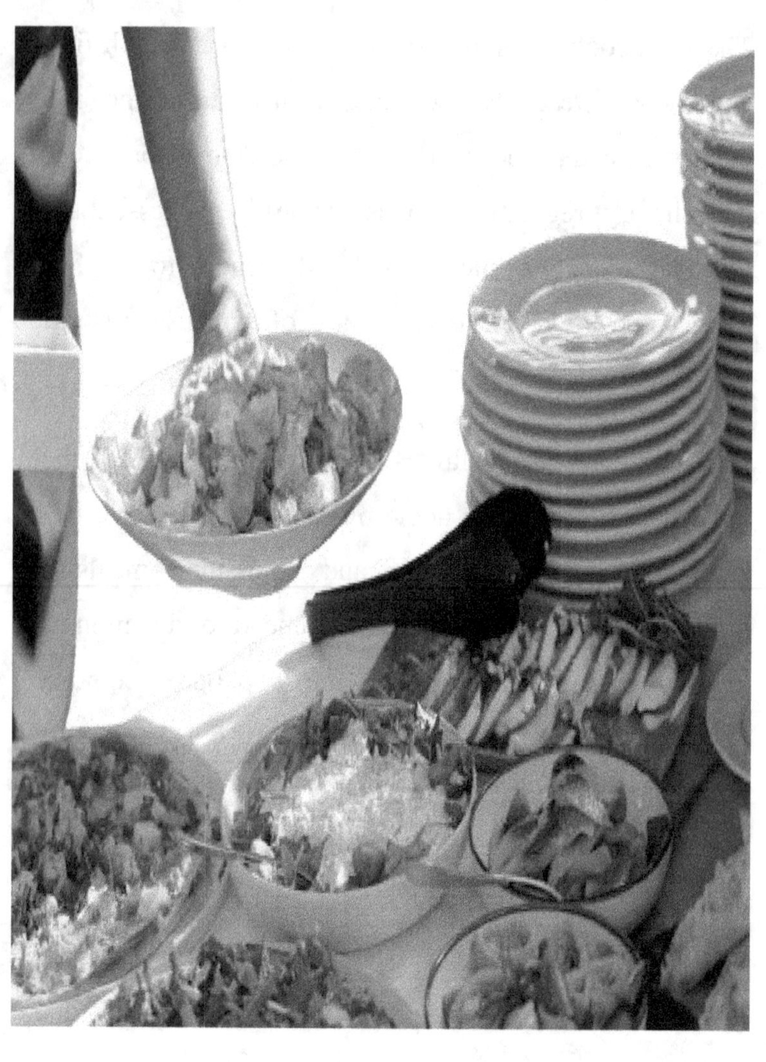

   The Flavorful Hypertension Diet Cookbook

Chapter 1: Understanding High Blood Pressure

Basic Information

Approximately Hypertension:

Hypertension, generally referred to as excessive blood strain, is a chronic clinical circumstance characterised via multiplied blood stress ranges inside the arteries.

The pressure exerted via the blood against the walls of the arteries is better than normal, putting an increased strain at the coronary heart. Hypertension is frequently referred to as a "silent killer" due to the fact it may increase over years without substantial symptoms, yet it poses extreme fitness dangers.

The two primary varieties of high blood pressure are number one (essential) high blood pressure, with out a identifiable purpose, and secondary hypertension, which ends up from an underlying health condition. Understanding the fundamentals of hypertension is vital for adopting preventative measures and way of life adjustments to control and manage blood stress correctly.

What Is High Blood Pressure?

High blood strain, or high blood pressure, is a medical circumstance characterized through multiplied blood pressure levels inside the arteries. The blood stress is the pressure of blood pushing in opposition to the walls of the arteries, and when this force is continuously excessive, it could lead to various health problems.

"The Flavorful Hypertension Diet Cookbook" begins its exploration by using emphasizing the essential expertise of high blood strain. In a simplified context, hypertension occurs when the coronary heart has to paintings more difficult than ordinary to pump blood, resulting in improved pressure on the arterial partitions.

This cookbook delves into the nuances of blood stress, offering a basis for readers to realize the effect of nutritional choices on their cardiovascular health.

How Do I Know If I Have High Blood Pressure?

One of the number one concerns for individuals is knowing whether they've excessive blood strain. "The Flavorful Hypertension Diet Cookbook" addresses this question comprehensively, losing mild at the symptoms and signs which could suggest elevated blood stress.

 Readers are guided via the importance of regular blood strain monitoring and a way to interpret the readings. The cookbook emphasizes the importance of cognizance and encourages readers to take proactive measures in coping with their cardiovascular fitness.

By providing insights into self-monitoring strategies and the relevance of ordinary take a look at-ups, the cookbook empowers individuals to be proactive in addressing capability hypertension worries.

What Is Considered High Blood Pressure?

"The Flavorful Hypertension Diet Cookbook" meticulously breaks down the classifications of blood pressure stages. Understanding what's considered excessive blood strain is important for powerful management. The cookbook delves into the 2 important components of blood stress readings: systolic and diastolic.

It elaborates at the ordinary range and outlines the thresholds that signify high blood pressure. By imparting this precise facts, the cookbook equips readers with the knowledge to identify when their blood strain falls outside the wholesome range.

This know-how serves as a foundation for the nutritional hints and recipes later added within the cookbook, emphasizing a holistic technique to high blood pressure management.

How Common Is High Blood Pressure?

The prevalence of high blood strain is a vital component mentioned in "The Flavorful Hypertension Diet Cookbook." The cookbook recognizes the big impact of high blood pressure on a worldwide scale. It highlights the alarming data surrounding the situation, emphasizing that hypertension isn't an remoted issue however a pervasive fitness concern affecting hundreds of thousands of individuals global.

By addressing the commonality of high blood strain, the cookbook ambitions to resonate with a wide audience, fostering a feel of community and shared duty in combating this generic fitness difficulty.

Symptoms Of High Blood Pressure

While hypertension is often called a "silent killer" due to its asymptomatic nature, "The Flavorful Hypertension Diet Cookbook" recognizes that some people may additionally experience symptoms. The cookbook affords an in-depth exploration of the diffused and frequently ignored signs and symptoms which can imply increased blood stress. By elucidating signs and symptoms such as complications, dizziness, and blurred vision, the cookbook encourages readers to be vigilant and are seeking for clinical attention in the event that they examine these caution symptoms. This emphasis on symptom recognition aligns with the cookbook's holistic method to high blood pressure management, integrating nutritional picks with ordinary fitness concerns.

Causes Of High Blood Pressure

"The Flavorful Hypertension Diet Cookbook" delves into the multifaceted causes of high blood stress, spotting that it is able to stem from a combination of genetic, way of life, and environmental elements.

The cookbook explores the role of dietary alternatives, sedentary existence, and pressure in contributing to multiplied blood strain levels. By elucidating those causes, the cookbook ambitions to empower readers to make informed lifestyle adjustments and dietary changes to manage and prevent high blood pressure. This comprehensive understanding of the basis causes of excessive blood stress units the degree for the cookbook's center focus on a flavorful and coronary heart-wholesome eating regimen as an fundamental thing of hypertension control.

Types Of High Blood Pressure:

Hypertension, or excessive blood pressure, is a medical situation characterized with the aid of increased blood strain levels. There are two important sorts of excessive blood strain: primary (vital) hypertension and secondary high blood pressure. Primary hypertension is the extra not unusual shape, accounting for approximately 90-ninety five% of cases.

It develops over time and has no identifiable purpose, often attributed to a combination of genetic and life-style elements. Secondary high blood pressure, on the other hand, is the end result of an underlying situation, which includes kidney disorder, hormonal issues, or certain medications. Understanding the form of high blood pressure is essential for tailoring an powerful treatment plan, whether thru way of life changes, remedy, or a combination of each.

Is High Blood Pressure Genetic

Genetics performs a substantial position in the improvement of high blood stress. While lifestyle factors like food plan and exercising contribute to high blood pressure, people with a family history of the situation are at a better threat.

Specific genetic elements can affect blood pressure law, such as genes related to salt sensitivity, blood vessel characteristic, and hormonal manipulate. Understanding the genetic aspect of hypertension is critical for each prevention and management. Individuals with a familial predisposition should be vigilant approximately life-style alternatives, together with a coronary heart-healthy weight loss plan and normal exercise, to mitigate the genetic hazard factors associated with high blood pressure.

Risk Factors For High Blood Pressure:

Several threat factors make contributions to the development of high blood stress, and understanding them is vital for powerful prevention and control. Lifestyle factors, consisting of a food regimen excessive in sodium, low potassium intake, sedentary conduct, and excessive alcohol intake, can extensively increase the hazard.

Other chance factors include age, as blood stress has a tendency to upward push with age, and race, with African Americans being greater susceptible. Obesity, stress, and smoking are additional modifiable chance factors that play a function in hypertension. By addressing these chance elements thru life-style modifications and early intervention, people can reduce their chance of growing excessive blood stress and its related complications.

Complications Of High Blood Pressure:

Uncontrolled excessive blood stress can lead to extreme complications, affecting various organs and structures inside the body. One of the most common headaches is cardiovascular ailment, inclusive of coronary heart attacks and strokes. Hypertension puts multiplied strain at the heart and blood vessels, main to damage over the years. It also can result in kidney ailment, because the kidneys are in particular sensitive to changes in blood pressure. Additionally, hypertension can purpose vision issues, peripheral artery disease, and cognitive decline.

Managing blood strain efficiently is vital to stopping these complications and preserving overall health. Regular tracking, adherence to treatment plans, and a healthy way of life are key additives of stopping the devastating results of out of control high blood pressure.

Diagnosis And Tests:

Diagnosing excessive blood strain involves measuring blood pressure levels the usage of a sphygmomanometer. The readings include numbers: systolic pressure (the strain while the coronary heart beats) and diastolic strain (the pressure whilst the coronary heart is at relaxation). A normal blood stress analyzing is commonly round a hundred and twenty/eighty mm Hg. Multiple readings may be taken over time to establish a analysis, as blood strain can range. Additionally, diverse assessments can be carried out to identify underlying reasons or check the impact of high blood pressure on organs.

These assessments may additionally include blood exams, urine assessments, electrocardiograms (ECGs or EKGs), and imaging studies like ultrasounds or CT scans. Accurate diagnosis is vital for growing a tailor-made treatment plan that addresses the unique wishes of the man or woman, whether or not through way of life adjustments, medicinal drugs, or a aggregate of each.

The Impact Of Diet On Blood Pressure:

Diet performs a pivotal function in handling high blood pressure, and "The Flavorful Hypertension Diet Cookbook" acknowledges this connection. Certain ingredients can make a contribution to accelerated blood strain, at the same time as others may additionally help lower it.

The cookbook likely emphasizes the importance of a balanced and heart-healthful weight loss program rich in culmination, veggies, lean proteins, and whole grains. The inclusion of precise nutrients like potassium, calcium, and magnesium, acknowledged for his or her blood pressure-regulating houses, is in all likelihood a key awareness. Additionally, the cookbook might also provide insights into the detrimental outcomes of immoderate sodium intake, a prime contributor to high blood pressure. Adopting a weight loss program that aligns with these ideas now not most effective aids in blood pressure management however additionally promotes general cardiovascular fitness.

Statistics And Facts To Emphasize The Prevalence Of Hypertension:

To underscore the urgency of addressing high blood pressure, it's miles vital to delve into applicable statistics and information. Hypertension is a worldwide health trouble affecting hundreds of thousands of humans, and its occurrence is progressively increasing.

According to the World Health Organization (WHO), an expected 1.13 billion human beings worldwide suffer from high blood pressure. In the US on my own, nearly half of of all adults are stricken by this condition. Shockingly, handiest about one in four people with high blood pressure have their condition below manage, highlighting the want for expanded attention and powerful control techniques. The impact of hypertension extends beyond character fitness, contributing notably to the worldwide burden of cardiovascular diseases.

The cookbook probably makes use of those information to emphasize the full-size nature of high blood pressure and the vital for individuals to adopt way of life adjustments, which include dietary changes, to shrink its prevalence.

In conclusion, "The Flavorful Hypertension Diet Cookbook" serves as an academic aid, offering vital records about high blood pressure, highlighting the tremendous have an effect on of weight-reduction plan on blood stress, and leveraging facts and statistics to underscore the worldwide occurrence of this health challenge. By delving into those components, people advantage a complete know-how of the significance of nutritional picks in managing high blood pressure and selling cardiovascular nicely-being.

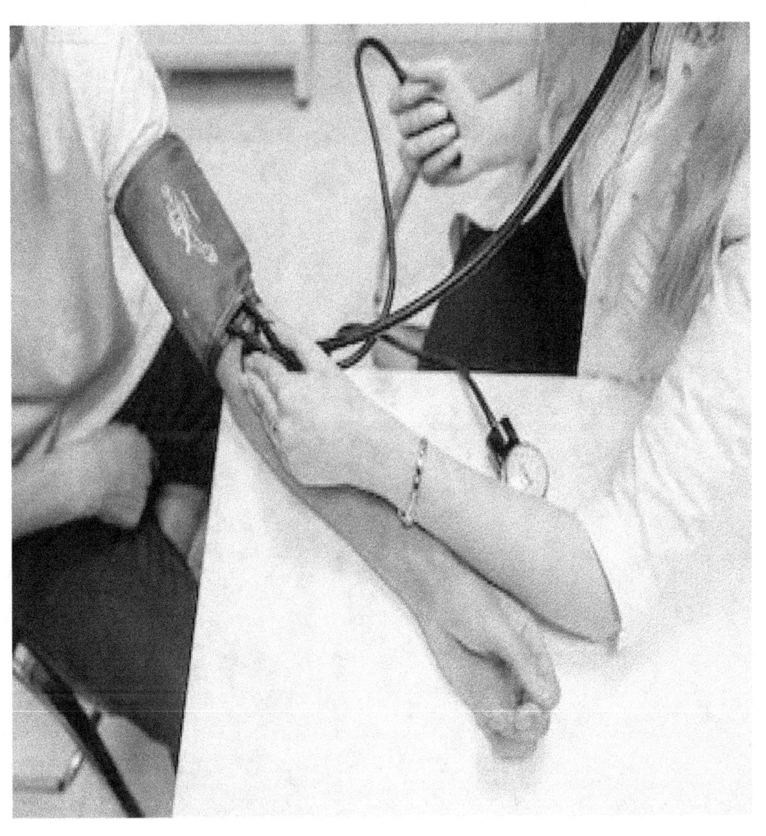

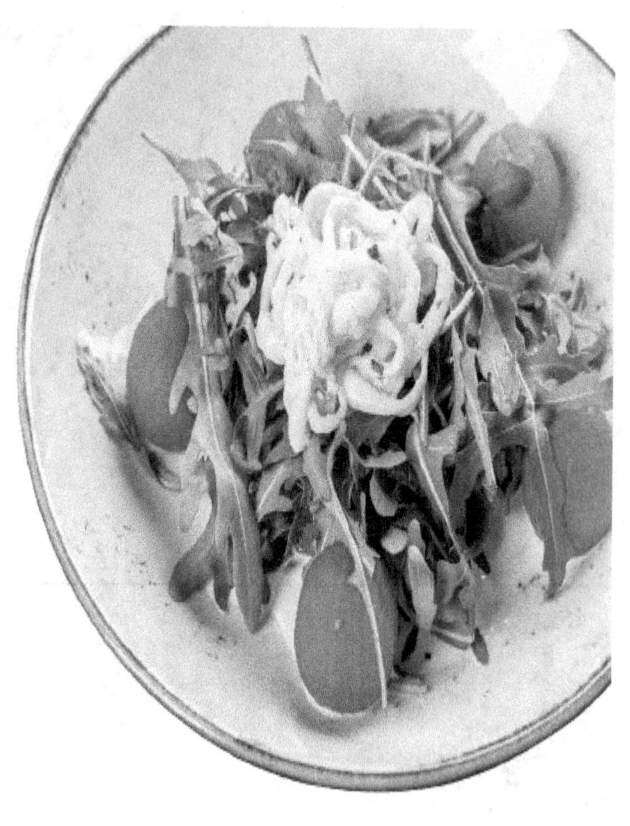

Chapter 2: The Science Behind The Flavors

Nutrients And Blood Pressure:

In the realm of hypertension management, know-how the pivotal function of key vitamins is paramount. The human frame operates as a complicated gadget where numerous vitamins play distinct roles in preserving physiological equilibrium. In the context of blood stress law, nutrients which include potassium, calcium, magnesium, and fiber grow to be protagonists.

Potassium, as an instance, orchestrates a sensitive stability with the aid of counteracting the sodium-brought on increase in blood stress. It helps vasodilation, reducing the strain on arterial walls. Calcium is involved in clean muscle contraction, influencing blood vessel tone. Magnesium, on the other hand, reveals vasodilatory consequences and aids within the right functioning of enzymes that modify blood pressure. Fiber, determined abundantly in end result, greens, and complete grains, contributes to decrease blood pressure by using promoting heart fitness and decreasing levels of cholesterol.

Delving into the difficult technology behind these nutrients, it becomes glaring that their affect extends beyond simplistic associations. For example, potassium's effect on blood stress hinges on its potential to negate the hypertensive consequences of sodium.

Sodium, regularly connected with accelerated blood stress, activates fluid retention and increases the volume of blood inside the arteries. Potassium intervenes by using facilitating the excretion of sodium via urine, attenuating its hypertensive impact. Furthermore, the vasodilatory effects of magnesium and calcium contribute to comfortable blood vessels, selling optimal blood flow.

Understanding the nuanced interplay of those vitamins equips people with the know-how to make knowledgeable dietary selections for effective high blood pressure control.

The Science Behind How Certain Ingredients Can Positively Affect Blood Pressure:

The fascinating science in the back of how particular elements wield have an effect on over blood pressure is a charming aspect of the hypertensive eating regimen. Certain culinary components stand out for his or her capability to not most effective tantalize flavor buds however also function allies in the conflict towards hypertension. Garlic, as an instance, has been a topic of clinical scrutiny for its ability antihypertensive houses. Allicin, a compound derived from garlic, is believed to loosen up blood vessels and reduce blood strain. Similarly, omega-3 fatty acids located in fatty fish like salmon and mackerel exhibit anti inflammatory and vasodilatory results, fostering a cardiovascular environment conducive to wholesome blood stress ranges.

Moreover, the inclusion of antioxidants-wealthy substances, significantly in end result and greens, contributes to blood stress regulation. Antioxidants combat oxidative strain, a aspect implicated in arterial stiffness and high blood pressure. Berries, spinach, and kale, encumbered with antioxidants like flavonoids and polyphenols, exemplify the dietary artillery available in a hypertensive-pleasant kitchen. Exploring the molecular intricacies, these antioxidants scavenge unfastened radicals, mitigating their unfavourable effect on blood vessels and ensuring a conducive surroundings for blood stress upkeep

In the labyrinth of scientific revelations, it's far fascinating to witness the emergence of spices along with turmeric and cinnamon as unsung heroes in the fight in opposition to high blood pressure. Curcumin, the lively compound in turmeric, well-knownshows anti-inflammatory and antioxidant homes, probably contributing to blood strain modulation. Cinnamon, with its specific taste profile, has been linked to improved arterial characteristic and decreased blood stress, presenting a palatable addition to hypertensive diets.

unraveling the science behind the flavors in "The Flavorful Hypertension Diet Cookbook" unveils a captivating narrative of nutrients and ingredients converging to create a symphony of flavor and health. The careful curation of recipes, informed by clinical insights, transforms the culinary experience into a healing journey for people searching for to manipulate hypertension via the artistry of nutrients.

The Science Behind The Flavors: Specific Herbs And Spices Known For Their Cardiovascular Benefits

The inclusion of unique herbs and spices in "The Flavorful Hypertension Diet Cookbook" isn't simply for culinary delight; it is a strategic preference rooted in the technology of cardiovascular fitness. One prominent herb renowned for its cardiovascular advantages is garlic. Scientifically, garlic consists of allicin, a compound that has been linked to decreasing blood pressure by using enjoyable blood vessels and promoting vasodilation. Additionally, garlic exhibits anti-inflammatory residences that contribute to universal coronary heart fitness. The inclusion of garlic within the cookbook no longer handiest enhances the flavor of the dishes however additionally aligns with the purpose of promoting a coronary heart-healthy food regimen.

Another noteworthy addition is turmeric, a spice celebrated for its lively factor, curcumin. The clinical community has significantly studied curcumin and set up its anti inflammatory and antioxidant houses. In the context of cardiovascular health, turmeric has been associated with stepped forward endothelial feature and decreased oxidative pressure, each critical elements in maintaining most effective blood strain levels. The cookbook's integration of turmeric underscores a dedication to now not only tantalizing flavor buds but additionally nurturing a food regimen that supports heart well-being.

Moving on to the world of spices, cinnamon emerges as a celeb factor with profound implications for blood strain regulation. Cinnamon consists of cinnamaldehyde, which has established potential in lowering blood stress by means of improving vasodilation and improving blood vessel function. Moreover, cinnamon has been linked to lowering levels of cholesterol, any other crucial aspect of cardiovascular health. The cookbook's incorporation of cinnamon is a testament to its determination to flavor enhancement coupled with a scientific expertise of how particular spices make a contribution to a heart-friendly food plan.

Basil, a fragrant herb frequently related to Italian delicacies, reveals its area within the cookbook because of its cardiovascular blessings. Rich in flavonoids and crucial oils, basil possesses anti inflammatory and anti-oxidative properties that contribute to the preservation of healthy blood pressure degrees.

Studies have indicated that basil extracts may additionally help relax blood vessels, promoting improved flow and mitigating hypertension. By together with basil in the recipes, the cookbook no longer best imparts a satisfying flavor but also harnesses the capacity fitness blessings embedded in this versatile herb.

In precis, the choice of precise herbs and spices in "The Flavorful Hypertension Diet Cookbook" isn't always arbitrary; it's far a planned fusion of culinary artistry and clinical expertise. Garlic, turmeric, cinnamon, and basil, each celebrated for his or her specific cardiovascular advantages, make a contribution no longer best to the palatability of the dishes but also to the overarching purpose of selling heart fitness. By imparting a comprehensive exploration of the technological know-how behind those flavors, the cookbook empowers readers to make knowledgeable choices for his or her cardiovascular nicely-being, reworking ordinary

Equipment Essential For Cooking Healthful, Flavorful Food

Setting up a high blood pressure-friendly kitchen begins with obtaining the crucial tools important for cooking healthful and flavorful meals. These tools play a vital role in promoting a balanced and nutritious weight loss program tailor-made to manipulate blood strain stages effectively.

 A well-ready kitchen now not best simplifies the cooking procedure however additionally encourages the incorporation of clean, whole elements that make contributions to overall cardiovascular fitness.

First and main, making an investment in high-quality knives is paramount. A sharp set of knives now not best expedites the practise procedure however additionally ensures precision in reducing fruits, greens, and lean proteins. Properly cut components permit for even cooking and beautify the overall presentation of dishes, making the culinary experience more exciting.

 Precision in knife paintings is especially essential whilst handling unique dietary necessities, inclusive of decreasing sodium content material or controlling element sizes to hold a heart-healthy weight loss program.

In addition to knives, selecting the proper cookware is important for a hypertension-pleasant kitchen. Opting for non-stick pans reduces the need for immoderate cooking oils, minimizing needless fat intake. Additionally, the usage of cookware crafted from materials along with stainless steel or ceramic facilitates maintain the integrity of meals flavors with out compromising on fitness.

Non-reactive cookware ensures that acidic ingredients, frequently popular in heart-healthful recipes, do no longer leach dangerous substances into the meals, preserving both flavor and nutritional value.

Furthermore, incorporating innovative kitchen gadgets could make meal coaching greater green and exciting. Devices like blenders and meals processors aid in creating clean sauces, soups, and dips without the want for brought salt or unhealthy fats.

These gear empower people to test with various herbs and spices, adding depth and complexity to dishes at the same time as adhering to high blood pressure nutritional pointers. Moreover, investing in a virtual kitchen scale facilitates specific component control, an vital issue of dealing with sodium and calorie consumption for people with high blood pressure.

A essential component of a high blood pressure-pleasant kitchen is a flexible and nicely-stocked pantry. Including coronary heart-healthful staples like complete grains, legumes, and a lot of herbs and spices guarantees that flavorful food may be created with minimal reliance on excessive-sodium processed elements. A properly-organized pantry also allows higher meal planning, making it less difficult to follow dietary guidelines and keep a wholesome ingesting habitual.

Lastly, it's essential to prioritize garage answers that assist the toughness of fresh produce. Refrigerators with ample space for end result, greens, and lean proteins permit people to inventory up on important ingredients, reducing the reliance on processed and convenience foods. Proper storage boxes, including glass or BPA-free plastic, keep meals freshness without compromising on safety. This emphasis on fresh, entire meals no longer simplest aligns with hypertension dietary guidelines but also contributes to an usual nutritious and pleasing culinary revel in.

In end, equipping a hypertension-friendly kitchen includes considerate consideration of the tools necessary for cooking wholesome and flavorful food. From precision knives to non-reactive cookware, progressive kitchen gadgets to a well-stocked pantry, every detail performs a essential role in selling heart-wholesome cooking practices. By making an investment in those gear and prioritizing fresh, complete elements, individuals can create a culinary surroundings that helps their adventure in the direction of coping with hypertension through scrumptious and nutritious food.

Comprehensive List Of Pantry Staples Suitable For A Hypertension-Friendly Diet:

Creating a hypertension-friendly kitchen begins with stocking it with the right pantry staples. These necessities no longer handiest upload taste on your dishes but additionally contribute to a coronary heart-healthful life-style. First and essential, emphasize entire grains which includes quinoa, brown rice, and entire wheat pasta.

These grains are wealthy in fiber, which allows regulate blood pressure. Opt for low-sodium canned goods like beans, tomatoes, and greens to decrease salt consumption. Incorporating quite a few herbs and spices, such as garlic, ginger, and turmeric, can decorate the flavor of your meals without the want for immoderate salt.

Choose coronary heart-wholesome oils like olive oil and avocado oil over saturated fats, promoting better cardiovascular health. Nuts and seeds, along with almonds, chia seeds, and flaxseeds, are incredible resources of omega-three fatty acids, which have been linked to decrease blood strain. Lastly, maintain a selection of canned or dried culmination without a added sugars for a herbal sweetness increase. This complete list ensures that your kitchen is properly-ready for preparing flavorful and hypertension-friendly food.

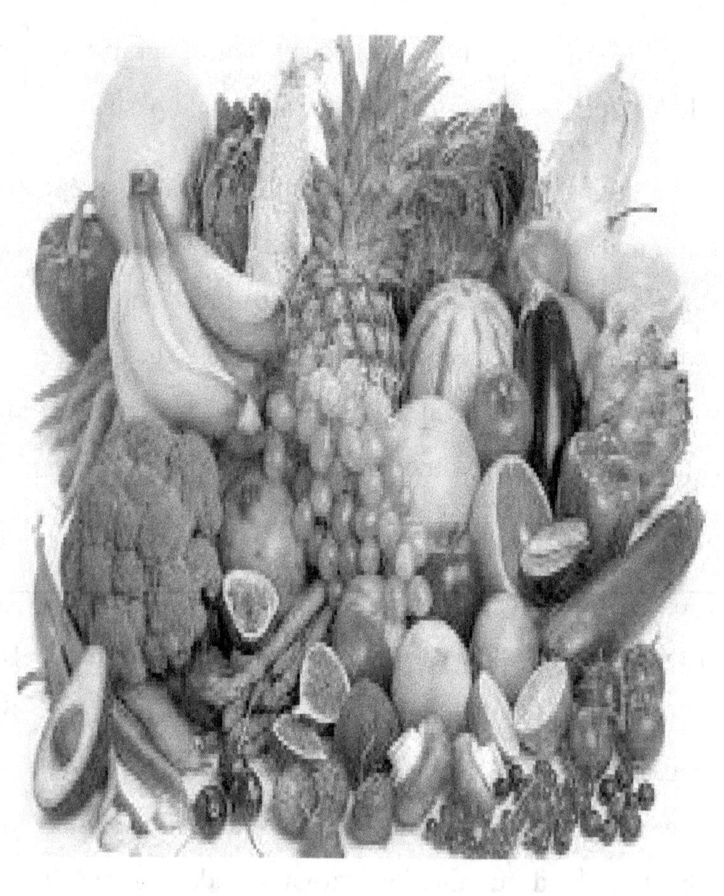

Chapter 3: Building Flavorful Foundations

Tips On Smart Grocery Shopping For Heart-Healthy Ingredients:

Navigating the grocery store with a focus on coronary heart-healthful substances is important for people handling hypertension. Begin by means of making plans your food and developing an in depth purchasing listing to keep away from impulsive purchases and keep on with a nutritious weight loss plan.

Prioritize fresh produce, consisting of leafy veggies, colorful vegetables, and end result, as they may be wealthy in nutrients, minerals, and antioxidants that aid coronary heart health. When choosing protein assets, choose lean alternatives like skinless hen, fish, and legumes. Check labels for sodium content material, choosing low-sodium or no-delivered-salt variations of canned goods, sauces, and condiments. Explore the fringe of the grocery save, wherein sparkling and minimally processed meals are commonly located, whilst fending off the middle aisles that frequently incorporate processed and excessive-sodium products. Embrace whole grains through choosing whole wheat bread, brown rice, and oats over delicate alternatives. Consider incorporating dairy or dairy options with decrease fat content to reduce saturated fat consumption.

Finally, keep in mind of element sizes to keep a balanced weight loss plan and save you overeating. By following those suggestions, you could make knowledgeable selections throughout grocery purchasing, fostering a coronary heart-healthy kitchen that helps high blood pressure management.

Building Flavorful Foundations: Simple, Versatile Recipes For Sauces, Broths, And Dressings

Creating a high blood pressure-pleasant food regimen that is each delicious and health-conscious necessitates the development of flavorful foundations thru simple, versatile recipes for sauces, broths, and dressings. These culinary elements no longer most effective add a burst of flavor to food but also function the backbone for a various range of dishes. In the realm of sauces, the emphasis lies on concocting flavorful blends that raise the overall dining enjoy without compromising on fitness.

A prime instance would be a tomato-based sauce enriched with garlic, herbs, and a dash of olive oil, presenting a robust taste profile even as maintaining a low sodium content material important for high blood pressure control. Versatility is key in making sure those sauces may be seamlessly incorporated into diverse dishes, along with entire grain pasta or lean protein alternatives.

Moving on to broths, their significance cannot be overstated within the context of a high blood pressure-conscious diet. Broths not best shape the bottom for soups however also contribute to the depth of flavor in severa recipes.

The attention right here is on crafting broths with a foundation of nutrient-dense veggies, herbs, and lean proteins. A vegetable broth, as an instance, may characteristic ingredients like carrots, celery, and onions, enhancing the general taste without relying on immoderate salt. By incorporating broths into food, individuals can enjoy flavorful and satisfying dishes at the same time as adhering to nutritional suggestions aimed at coping with high blood pressure.

Dressings play a essential role in reworking everyday salads into delectable, heart-healthful culinary delights. The cookbook locations a sturdy emphasis on the use of fresh, entire substances in dressings to decorate flavor with out compromising on dietary price.

A conventional vinaigrette, as an example, may feature greater virgin olive oil, balsamic vinegar, and a medley of herbs and spices. This not simplest imparts a burst of taste to salads but also contributes beneficial vitamins. The integration of entire elements ensures that dressings are not handiest delicious but also assist standard fitness, a cornerstone of the Flavorful Hypertension Diet Cookbook.

Balancing Flavors:

Balancing flavors is a essential factor of creating a hypertensive-friendly food plan this is both fitness-conscious and delicious. In "The Flavorful Hypertension Diet Cookbook," the emphasis on balancing flavors serves as a vital guide for readers looking for to decorate their culinary stories while adhering to dietary regulations. The number one undertaking lies in mitigating the reliance on extra salt and bad fat, which might be usually associated with traditional flavor enhancements. To attain this sensitive balance, the cookbook presents a complete method that entails incorporating quite a few herbs, spices, and other natural taste enhancers.

One key approach in balancing flavors is the artful use of herbs and spices. These substances no longer simplest add depth and complexity to dishes but additionally make contributions a plethora of fitness blessings.

The cookbook educates readers on the extraordinary taste profiles of herbs and spices, empowering them to make knowledgeable choices based on non-public options and nutritional desires. For instance, the inclusion of aromatic herbs like basil, thyme, and rosemary can impart savory notes to dishes, lowering the need for excessive salt. Meanwhile, spices consisting of cumin, turmeric, and cinnamon no longer best raise the flavor but also provide antioxidant and anti-inflammatory residences, promoting universal cardiovascular health.

Furthermore, the cookbook explores alternative assets of umami, the 5th basic taste, beyond the standard reliance on sodium-weighted down substances. Umami rich ingredients, together with mushrooms, tomatoes, and seaweed, are added as flavorful substitutes that enhance taste without compromising fitness. The cookbook guides readers via incorporating those ingredients into their recipes, fostering a palate that appreciates the nuanced interaction of flavors.

In addition to herbs, spices, and umami-wealthy foods, the cookbook delves into the strategic use of healthful fat to reap flavor balance. Avocado, olive oil, and nuts come to be culinary allies, presenting richness and satiety to food without resorting to unhealthy saturated fats. By emphasizing those alternatives, the cookbook empowers readers to make conscious alternatives that prioritize coronary heart fitness at the same time as savoring the indulgence of flavorful dishes.

The concept of flavor balancing extends past man or woman ingredients to the general composition of food. Readers are advocated to discover the synergy of various tastes—sweet, salty, bitter, sour, and umami—within a single dish.

This holistic approach no longer simplest enhances the gustatory revel in however also diminishes the need for excessive seasoning. The cookbook presents realistic suggestions and pattern recipes that exhibit how to obtain this stability, guiding readers toward culinary mastery while keeping their hypertensive issues in thoughts.

Ultimately, the emphasis on balancing flavors in "The Flavorful Hypertension Diet Cookbook" represents a transformative culinary adventure. It empowers readers to disencumber themselves from the shackles of excessive salt and bad fat, paving the manner for a colourful, diverse, and heart-healthy gastronomic experience.

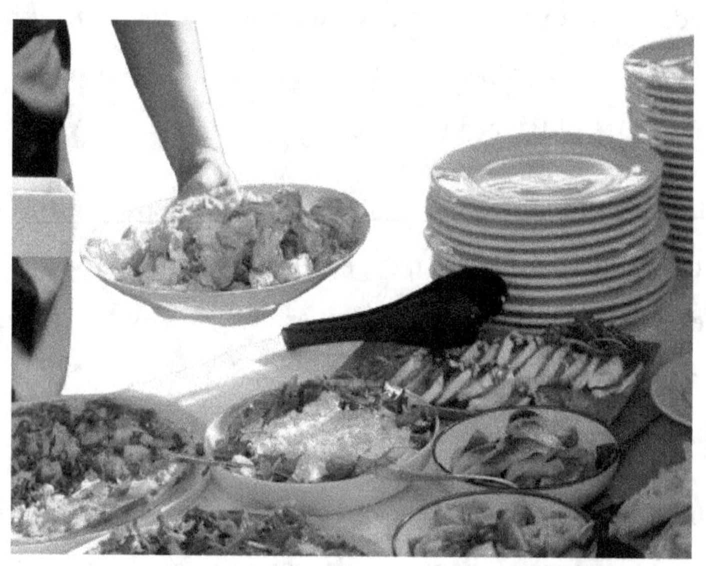

Chapter 4: 7 Days Meal Plan For Hypertension

Day 1:

Breakfast:

• Oatmeal with sliced bananas and a sprinkle of chia seeds.

• Green tea or black espresso (unsweetened).

Lunch:

• Grilled bird breast with quinoa.

• Steamed broccoli and carrots.

• Mixed green salad with olive oil and lemon dressing.

Snack:

• Greek yogurt with fresh berries.

Dinner:

- Baked salmon with lemon and herbs.

- Brown rice.

- Asparagus sautéed with garlic.

Day 2:

Breakfast:

- Whole grain toast with avocado.

- Poached eggs.

- Fresh orange juice (unsweetened).

Lunch:

- Lentil soup.

- Whole grain roll.

- Mixed vegetable salad.

Snack:

- Handful of almonds.

Dinner:

- Turkey stir-fry with colorful bell peppers and broccoli.

- Quinoa.

Day 3:

Breakfast:

- Smoothie with spinach, banana, berries, and occasional-fats yogurt.

Lunch:

- Chickpea salad with cherry tomatoes, cucumber, and feta cheese.

- Whole grain pita.

Snack:

- Carrot and cucumber sticks with hummus.

Dinner:

- Grilled shrimp with lemon and garlic.

- Sweet potato wedges.

- Steamed green beans.

Day 4:

Breakfast:

- Whole grain cereal with skim milk.

- Orange slices.

Lunch:

- Grilled vegetable wrap with whole grain tortilla.

- Quinoa salad.

Snack:

- Apple slices with almond butter.

Dinner:

- Baked cod with herbs.

- Brown rice.

- Roasted Brussels sprouts.

Day 5:

Breakfast:

- Greek yogurt parfait with granola and blended berries.

Lunch:

- Spinach and feta-stuffed fowl breast.

- Quinoa.

- Mixed green salad.

Snack:

- A small bunch of grapes.

Dinner:

- Stir-fried tofu with broccoli and snow peas.

- Brown rice.

Day 6:

Breakfast:

• Whole grain bagel with smoked salmon and cream cheese.

• Sliced tomatoes.

Lunch:

• Black bean and vegetable burrito bowl with brown rice.

• Salsa and guacamole.

Snack:

• Cottage cheese with pineapple chunks.

Dinner:

• Grilled chicken skewers with zucchini and cherry tomatoes.

• Quinoa.

Day 7:

Breakfast:

- Smoothie with kale, banana, pineapple, and coconut water.

Lunch:

- Whole grain pasta with tomato and vegetable sauce.

- Mixed green salad.

Snack:

- Handful of walnuts.

Dinner:

- Baked tilapia with lemon and herbs.

- Sweet potato mash.

- Steamed asparagus.

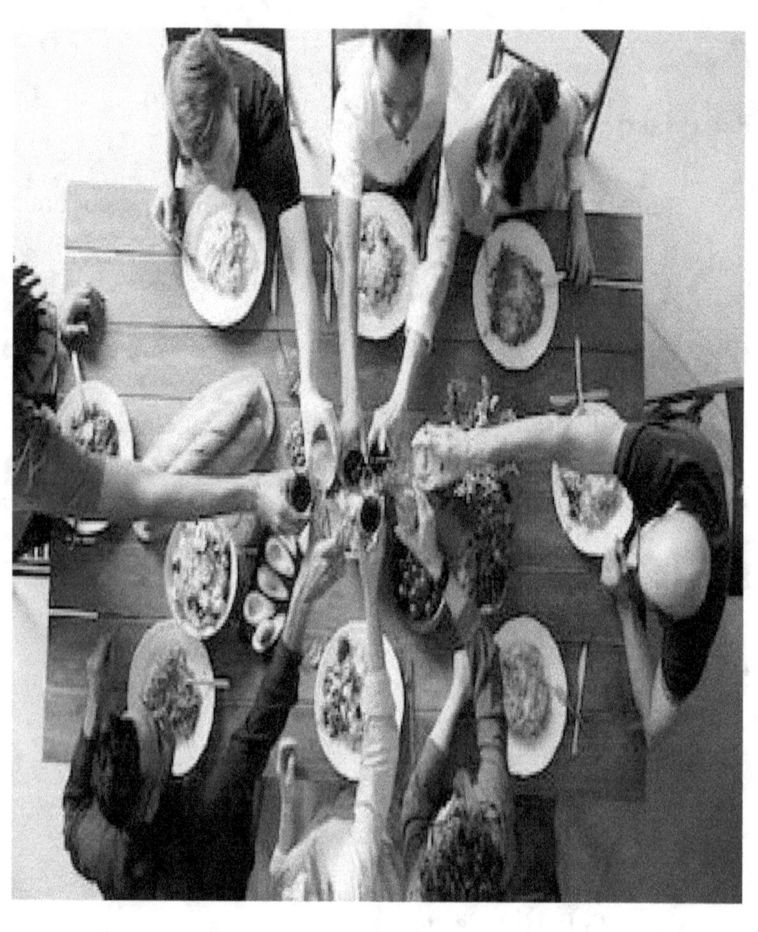

Chapter 5: Hypertension Recipe

Breakfast

1. Oatmeal and Berry Bliss Bowl

Introduction:

Start your day proper with a heart-wholesome breakfast that allows manage hypertension. This Oatmeal and Berry Bliss Bowl is wealthy in fiber, antioxidants, and potassium, promoting usual cardiovascular fitness.

Ingredients:

- half of cup rolled oats

- 1 cup almond milk (unsweetened)

- 1/2 cup blended berries (blueberries, strawberries, raspberries)

- 1 tablespoon chia seeds

- 1 tablespoon honey

- 1/4 teaspoon cinnamon

- half of banana, sliced

- 1 tablespoon chopped walnuts

Preparation Method:

1.   In a saucepan, integrate rolled oats and almond milk. Cook over medium warmness, stirring every so often, until the oats are tender.

2.   Mix inside the chia seeds, honey, and cinnamon. Stir well and cook dinner for an extra 2-three mins.

3.   Remove from heat and transfer the oatmeal to a bowl.

4.   Top with mixed berries, banana slices, and chopped walnuts.

5.   Enjoy a wholesome breakfast that supports heart fitness.

Prep Time: 10 minutes

2. Avocado And Tomato Breakfast Wrap

Introduction:

Kick start your day with this delicious Avocado and Tomato Breakfast Wrap, packed with vitamins to assist modify blood pressure. Avocado provides wholesome fats, while tomatoes contribute potassium and antioxidants.

Ingredients:

*   1 complete wheat tortilla

*   half of avocado, mashed

*   1 medium tomato, diced

*   2 eggs, scrambled

*   1/4 cup black beans (canned, drained, and rinsed)

- 1 tablespoon sparkling cilantro, chopped

- Salt and pepper to taste

- Hot sauce (non-compulsory)

Preparation Method:

1.   Warm the whole wheat tortilla in a dry skillet over medium warmth.

2.   Spread mashed avocado at the tortilla, leaving area around the rims.

3.   In the equal skillet, scramble the eggs till simply cooked. Season with salt and pepper.

4.   Layer the scrambled eggs, diced tomatoes, black beans, and sparkling cilantro over the avocado.

5.   Optional: Drizzle with warm sauce for an extra kick.

6.   Fold the sides of the tortilla in and roll it up right into a wrap.

7. Slice in 1/2 and serve straight away.

Prep Time: 15 minutes

Lunch

Recipe 1: Grilled Salmon Salad With Lemon-Dill Dressing

Introduction:

Elevate your lunch with this heart-healthful grilled salmon salad. Packed with omega-three fatty acids and nutrient-wealthy vegetables, this dish is ideal for the ones managing high blood pressure.

Ingredients:

*   2 salmon fillets

*   four cups combined vegetables (spinach, arugula, and kale)

- 1 cup cherry tomatoes, halved

- 1 cucumber, sliced

- 1/four crimson onion, thinly sliced

- 2 tablespoons olive oil

- 1 tablespoon clean lemon juice

- 1 teaspoon Dijon mustard

- 1 tablespoon clean dill, chopped

- Salt and pepper to flavor

Preparation Method:

1. Preheat the grill to medium-high warmth.

2. Season the salmon fillets with salt and pepper.

3. Grill the salmon for four-five minutes per side or until it flakes effortlessly with a fork.

4. In a big bowl, toss the combined greens, cherry tomatoes, cucumber, and pink onion.

5.   In a small bowl, whisk collectively olive oil, lemon juice, Dijon mustard, fresh dill, salt, and pepper to create the dressing.

6.   Place the grilled salmon on top of the salad and drizzle with the lemon-dill dressing.

7.   Serve without delay and enjoy a delicious, hypertension-pleasant lunch.

Prep Time: 20 minutes

Recipe 2: Quinoa and Vegetable Stir-Fry

Introduction:

For a satisfying and high blood pressure-pleasant lunch, do that quinoa and vegetable stir-fry. Packed with fiber, protein, and colorful greens, it is a delectable manner to guide heart fitness.

Ingredients:

*   1 cup quinoa, rinsed

- 2 cups broccoli florets

- 1 bell pepper, thinly sliced

- 1 carrot, julienned

- 1 cup snap peas, trimmed

- 3 tablespoons low-sodium soy sauce

- 1 tablespoon sesame oil

- 1 tablespoon rice vinegar

- 1 teaspoon ginger, minced

- 2 cloves garlic, minced

- 2 inexperienced onions, sliced

- 1 tablespoon sesame seeds (non-compulsory)

Preparation Method:

1. Cook quinoa in line with bundle instructions and set apart.

2.   In a large skillet or wok, warmness sesame oil over medium-excessive warmness.

3.   Add ginger and garlic, sauté for 1-2 minutes until fragrant.

4.   Add broccoli, bell pepper, carrot, and snap peas to the skillet. Stir-fry for 4-five minutes till greens are crisp-smooth.

5.   In a small bowl, whisk together soy sauce and rice vinegar. Pour over the greens and toss to coat frivolously.

6.   Add cooked quinoa to the skillet, stirring to combine with the vegetables.

7.   Garnish with sliced inexperienced onions and sesame seeds if preferred.

8.   Serve right now for a healthy, high blood pressure-pleasant lunch.

Prep Time: 30 minutes

Dinner

Recipe 1: Grilled Salmon With Garlic Spinach And Quinoa

Introduction:

This heart-healthful dinner is designed to support individuals dealing with high blood pressure. Grilled salmon, wealthy in omega-3 fatty acids, takes center degree along garlic-infused spinach and protein-packed quinoa, developing a scrumptious and nutritious meal.

Ingredients:

- 2 salmon fillets

- 2 cups sparkling spinach

- 1 cup quinoa

- three cloves garlic, minced

- 1 lemon, juiced

- 2 tablespoons olive oil

- Salt and pepper to flavor

Preparation:

1. Cook quinoa in step with package deal commands.

2. Season salmon fillets with salt, pepper, and a drizzle of olive oil. Grill for 4-5 mins on each facet or until cooked via.

3. In a pan, sauté minced garlic in olive oil until golden. Add fresh spinach and cook till wilted.

4. Serve grilled salmon over a mattress of cooked quinoa, crowned with garlic spinach. Drizzle with sparkling lemon juice.

Prep Time: Approximately 25 minutes.

Recipe 2: Mediterranean Chickpea Salad With Baked Chicken

Introduction:

This hypertension-friendly dinner functions a vibrant Mediterranean chickpea salad paired with baked chook breasts. Packed with fiber, antioxidants, and lean protein, this dish no longer simplest helps heart health but also delights the taste buds.

Ingredients:

- 2 boneless, skinless chook breasts

- 1 can (15 oz) chickpeas, tired and rinsed

- 1 cucumber, diced

- 1 cup cherry tomatoes, halved

- half purple onion, finely chopped

- 1/4 cup feta cheese, crumbled

- three tablespoons extra-virgin olive oil

- 2 tablespoons balsamic vinegar

- 1 teaspoon dried oregano

- Salt and pepper to flavor

Preparation:

1.   Preheat the oven to four hundred°F (200°C). Season bird breasts with salt, pepper, and dried oregano. Bake for 20-25 minutes or until cooked through.

2.   In a huge bowl, combine chickpeas, cucumber, cherry tomatoes, pink onion, and feta cheese.

3.   In a small bowl, whisk collectively olive oil and balsamic vinegar. Season with salt and pepper.

4.   Slice baked chook and serve over the Mediterranean chickpea salad. Drizzle the dressing over the top.

Prep Time: Approximately 30 minutes.

Snacks

Recipe 1: Avocado And Tomato Bruschetta

Introduction:

This high blood pressure-friendly snack combines the heart-healthy fats of avocados with the antioxidant-rich tomatoes, served on complete-grain toast for an delivered fiber increase. It's a delicious and pleasing choice that helps a balanced food regimen for the ones managing high blood pressure.

Ingredients:

- 1 ripe avocado, diced

- 1 cup cherry tomatoes, halved

- 2 tablespoons red onion, finely chopped

- 1 tablespoon fresh basil, chopped

- 1 tablespoon balsamic vinegar

- Salt and pepper to flavor

- 4 slices whole-grain bread, toasted

Preparation Method:

1. In a bowl, integrate diced avocado, cherry tomatoes, crimson onion, and fresh basil.

2. Drizzle balsamic vinegar over the mixture and lightly toss until components are lightly coated.

3. Season with salt and pepper to taste.

4. Spoon the avocado and tomato mixture onto the toasted complete-grain bread slices.

5. Serve immediately and enjoy this nutrient-packed bruschetta.

Prep Time: Approximately 15 minutes.

Recipe 2: Greek Yogurt And Berry Parfait

Introduction:

This delightful yogurt parfait isn't most effective scrumptious but additionally wealthy in potassium and low in sodium, making it an fantastic preference for individuals with hypertension. The combination of Greek yogurt and fresh berries presents a burst of flavor along side important vitamins for coronary heart health.

Ingredients:

•   1 cup plain Greek yogurt

•   1 cup mixed berries (strawberries, blueberries, raspberries)

•   2 tablespoons honey

•   1/four cup granola (low-sugar and coffee-sodium)

•   1 teaspoon chia seeds (non-compulsory)

Preparation Method:

1.   In a tumbler or bowl, layer half of the Greek yogurt at the bottom.

2.   Add a layer of mixed berries on top of the yogurt.

3.   Drizzle 1 tablespoon of honey over the berries.

4.   Sprinkle 1/2 of the granola on the berries.

5.   Repeat the layers with the final yogurt, berries, honey, and granola.

6.   Optionally, sprinkle chia seeds on top for a further nutritional raise.

7.   Refrigerate for a couple of minutes earlier than serving to allow flavors to meld.

Prep Time: Approximately 10 mins.

Recipe 1: Mediterranean Quinoa Salad With Grilled Salmon

Introduction:

Indulge in a heart-wholesome wilderness with this fresh Mediterranean Quinoa Salad proposing grilled salmon. Packed with nutrients, this dish isn't always simplest delicious but additionally useful for those dealing with hypertension.

Ingredients:

- 1 cup quinoa, rinsed

- 2 cups cherry tomatoes, halved

- 1 cucumber, diced

- half red onion, finely chopped

- 1/4 cup Kalamata olives, sliced

- four tablespoons feta cheese, crumbled

- 2 salmon fillets

- 2 tablespoons olive oil

- Juice of one lemon

- 2 teaspoons dried oregano

- Salt and pepper to taste

Preparation:

1.	Cook quinoa in step with package deal commands.

2.	Season salmon with olive oil, lemon juice, oregano, salt, and pepper. Grill till cooked through.

3.	In a huge bowl, combine cooked quinoa, cherry tomatoes, cucumber, pink onion, olives, and feta cheese.

4.	Flake grilled salmon into chew-sized portions and lightly fold into the salad.

5.	Drizzle with greater olive oil, if desired, and season to flavor.

6.   Serve immediately or refrigerate for a calming choice.

Prep Time: Approximately 30 minutes.

Recipe 2: Berry Parfait With Greek Yogurt And Almond Crunch

Introduction:

Satisfy your sweet cravings with this pleasant Berry Parfait, a high blood pressure-friendly dessert that combines the goodness of antioxidant-rich berries, creamy Greek yogurt, and a delightful almond crunch.

Ingredients:

•   2 cups combined berries (strawberries, blueberries, raspberries)

•   2 cups Greek yogurt

•   1/four cup honey

- 1 teaspoon vanilla extract

- half cup almonds, chopped

- 2 tablespoons honey (for almond crunch)

- Fresh mint leaves for garnish

Preparation:

1. In a bowl, mix Greek yogurt with honey and vanilla extract.

2. In serving glasses, layer Greek yogurt aggregate with mixed berries.

3. Repeat the layers till the glass is sort of complete, ending with a layer of berries on pinnacle.

4. In a pan, toast chopped almonds till golden. Add honey and stir until almonds are coated.

5. Sprinkle the almond crunch over the berry layers.

6. Garnish with sparkling mint leaves.

Prep Time: Approximately 20 minutes.

Smoothies

Smoothie Recipe 1: Berry Bliss Hypertension Buster

Introduction:

This pleasant Berry Bliss Hypertension Buster smoothie is packed with antioxidants and nutrients recognised to guide heart health. The combination of berries presents a burst of taste whilst selling lower blood stress.

Ingredients:

- 1 cup combined berries (blueberries, strawberries, raspberries)

- 1 medium banana

- half of cup spinach leaves

- 1/2 cup Greek yogurt

- 1 tablespoon chia seeds

- 1 cup almond milk

- Ice cubes (optionally available)

Preparation Method:

1.   Wash the berries and spinach very well.

2.   Peel and slice the banana.

3.   In a blender, integrate the mixed berries, banana slices, spinach leaves, Greek yogurt, chia seeds, and almond milk.

4.   Blend on high velocity until smooth and creamy.

5.   If favored, upload ice cubes and mix once more for a refreshing kick back.

6.   Pour into a tumbler and enjoy this nutrient-packed hypertension-busting smoothie!

Prep Time: Approximately 5 minutes

Smoothie Recipe 2: Green Goddess Hypertension Elixir

Introduction:

Elevate your coronary heart fitness with the Green Goddess Hypertension Elixir. This vibrant inexperienced smoothie is rich in potassium and magnesium, important minerals that contribute to blood pressure law.

Ingredients:

- 1 cup kale leaves, stems removed

- 1/2 cucumber, peeled and sliced

- half avocado

- half of cup pineapple chunks

- 1 tablespoon flaxseeds

- 1 tablespoon honey (elective for sweetness)

- 1 cup coconut water

- Ice cubes (elective)

Preparation Method:

1. Wash the kale leaves and cucumber very well.

2. Peel and pit the avocado.

3. In a blender, combine kale leaves, cucumber slices, avocado, pineapple chunks, flaxseeds, honey (if the use of), and coconut water.

4. Blend until the aggregate reaches a smooth consistency.

5. If you decide on a less warm smoothie, upload ice cubes and blend again.

6. Pour into a glass, and relish the Green Goddess Hypertension Elixir for a clean and heart-wholesome treat.

Prep Time: Approximately 7 mins

Conclusion

In the savory adventure through the pages of "The Flavorful Hypertension Diet Cookbook," we've got explored a world where fitness-aware picks harmonize seamlessly with tantalizing tastes. As we finish this culinary journey, permit's savor the essence of what makes this cookbook virtually exquisite.

This cookbook is not just a compilation of recipes; it's far a testament to the transformative energy of scrumptious, nutritious food. It effects proves that handling hypertension doesn't suggest sacrificing taste. Instead, it invitations you to embody a vibrant tapestry of components that now not handiest nurture your nicely-being however additionally indulge your taste buds in a symphony of tastes and aromas.

Beyond being an insignificant series of recipes, this cookbook stands as a culinary companion, a reliable manual on your adventure to higher fitness. It encapsulates the concept that wholesome eating isn't approximately deprivation; it's approximately a joyful birthday party of nourishment. The carefully crafted recipes inside those pages are a manifestation of a commitment to both flavor and well-being, a stability that elevates every meal to a delightful enjoy.

So, as you embark to your very own gastronomic day trip armed with these recipes, take into account that each dish is a step toward a healthier, more colourful you. Let this cookbook be your compass in the kitchen, guiding you to a world wherein high blood pressure management isn't always a compromise however an exploration of the diverse, scrumptious possibilities that lie in each meal.

In last, might also your culinary adventures be as wealthy as the flavors inside these pages, and might the path to a more fit life-style be paved with the pleasure of top meals. "The Flavorful Hypertension Diet Cookbook" is greater than a cookbook; it is an invitation to take pleasure in lifestyles, one delicious and coronary heart-healthful chew at a time. Cheers to a adventure of health and taste!

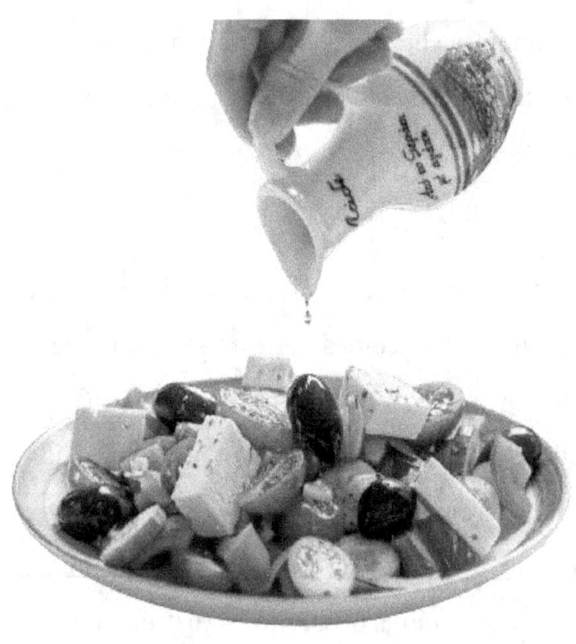

Meal planner journal for a week

Dates

Meal planner journal
for a week

	BREAKFAST MEAL	LUNCH	DINNER	SNACKS
MON				
TUE				
WED				
THU				
FRI				
SAT				
SUN				

NOTE

Shopping list

NOTE

Eat healthy food and you will be fine

Meal planner journal
for a week

	BREAKFAST MEAL	LUNCH	DINNER	SNACKS
MON				
TUE				
WED				
THU				
FRI				
SAT				
SUN				

NOTE

Shopping list

NOTE

Eat healthy food and you will be fine

Meal planner journal
for a week

	BREAKFAST MEAL	LUNCH	DINNER	SNACKS
MON				
TUE				
WED				
THU				
FRI				
SAT				
SUN				

NOTE

Shopping list

NOTE

Eat healthy food and you will be fine

Dates

	BREAKFAST MEAL	LUNCH	DINNER	SNACKS
MON				
TUE				
WED				
THU				
FRI				
SAT				
SUN				

NOTE

Shopping list

NOTE

Eat healthy food and you will be fine

| Dates |

Meal planner journal
for a week

	BREAKFAST MEAL	LUNCH	DINNER	SNACKS
MON				
TUE				
WED				
THU				
FRI				
SAT				
SUN				

NOTE   Shopping list   **NOTE**

Eat healthy food and you will be fine

Dates

	BREAKFAST MEAL	LUNCH	DINNER	SNACKS
MON				
TUE				
WED				
THU				
FRI				
SAT				
SUN				

NOTE Shopping list **NOTE**

Eat healthy food and you will be fine

Meal planner journal
for a week

	BREAKFAST MEAL	LUNCH	DINNER	SNACKS
MON				
TUE				
WED				
THU				
FRI				
SAT				
SUN				

NOTE

Shopping list

NOTE

Eat healthy food and you will be fine

Dates

	BREAKFAST MEAL	LUNCH	DINNER	SNACKS
MON				
TUE				
WED				
THU				
FRI				
SAT				
SUN				

NOTE

Shopping list

NOTE

Eat healthy food and you will be fine

Dates

	BREAKFAST MEAL	LUNCH	DINNER	SNACKS
MON				
TUE				
WED				
THU				
FRI				
SAT				
SUN				

NOTE   Shopping list   **NOTE**

Eat healthy food and you will be fine

Meal planner journal
for a week

	BREAKFAST MEAL	LUNCH	DINNER	SNACKS
MON				
TUE				
WED				
THU				
FRI				
SAT				
SUN				

NOTE   Shopping list   **NOTE**

Eat healthy food and you will be fine

Dates

	BREAKFAST MEAL	LUNCH	DINNER	SNACKS
MON				
TUE				
WED				
THU				
FRI				
SAT				
SUN				

NOTE

Shopping list

NOTE

Eat healthy food and you will be fine

Dates

	BREAKFAST MEAL	LUNCH	DINNER	SNACKS
MON				
TUE				
WED				
THU				
FRI				
SAT				
SUN				

NOTE

Shopping list

NOTE

Eat healthy food and you will be fine

Meal planner journal
for a week

	BREAKFAST MEAL	LUNCH	DINNER	SNACKS
MON				
TUE				
WED				
THU				
FRI				
SAT				
SUN				

NOTE

Shopping list

NOTE

Eat healthy food and you will be fine

Dates

	BREAKFAST MEAL	LUNCH	DINNER	SNACKS
MON				
TUE				
WED				
THU				
FRI				
SAT				
SUN				

NOTE

Shopping list

NOTE

Eat healthy food and you will be fine

Meal planner journal
for a week

	BREAKFAST MEAL	LUNCH	DINNER	SNACKS
MON				
TUE				
WED				
THU				
FRI				
SAT				
SUN				

NOTE

Shopping list

NOTE

Eat healthy food and you will be fine

Meal planner journal
for a week

	BREAKFAST MEAL	LUNCH	DINNER	SNACKS
MON				
TUE				
WED				
THU				
FRI				
SAT				
SUN				

NOTE

Shopping list

NOTE

Eat healthy food and you will be fine

Meal planner journal
for a week

	BREAKFAST MEAL	LUNCH	DINNER	SNACKS
MON				
TUE				
WED				
THU				
FRI				
SAT				
SUN				

NOTE   Shopping list   **NOTE**

Eat healthy food and you will be fine

Dates

	BREAKFAST MEAL	LUNCH	DINNER	SNACKS
MON				
TUE				
WED				
THU				
FRI				
SAT				
SUN				

NOTE

Shopping list

NOTE

Eat healthy food and you will be fine

Dates

	BREAKFAST MEAL	LUNCH	DINNER	SNACKS
MON				
TUE				
WED				
THU				
FRI				
SAT				
SUN				

NOTE

Shopping list

NOTE

Eat healthy food and you will be fine

Meal planner journal
for a week

	BREAKFAST MEAL	LUNCH	DINNER	SNACKS
MON				
TUE				
WED				
THU				
FRI				
SAT				
SUN				

NOTE   Shopping list   **NOTE**

Eat healthy food and you will be fine